DOS AND DON'TS OF RIDDING YOUR FACE OF ACNE PIMPLES

Discipline is the soul of an army. It takes discipline to succeed and achieve anything in life. Be it slimming down, obtaining another degree, winning a medal in a tournament, name it, discipline is it.

I believe you paid something for this information, therefore I believe you will make something out of it and not throw it into a corner of your library, allow it to lie on a shelf gathering dust or leave in a folder in computer until it gets infected with virus.

As said what you need is discipline to make what I am going to share with you work. A consistent and steadfast application of what I will share with you.

For it to work you will need

1.   Discipline

2.   Self-control

3.   Self-denial

I may take them one by one later or simply be laying emphasis on them, as we press on, but first let me share the information with you. That is why there is nothing like money back guarantee in this deal.

Here we go:

I am not sending you a drug, be it herbal or chemical but a simple dos and don'ts of how to rid your face of stubborn acne and pimples without any antiseptic soap, chemical or drugs. Something I have practised and experimented that worked for me. And which I have also verbally recommended to others with amazing Results within 2 months of their following the simple instructions.

Let us go to the don'ts first. Prevention has been proven times without number to be FAR better and cheaper than cure. But the beauty of what we are sharing here is it is both **preventive and curative.**

THE DON'TS

Acne and pimples thrives in an oily environment of an oily face.

The truth is that we all need a level of oil secreted and generated in our body to keep it smooth and keep it from dryness. Therefore oil lubricates the skin and body pores and keeps it smooth and beautiful.

But as the saying goes, too much of anything is bad. Where there is too much secretion and generation of it especially on the facial cavity, first, the face adopts a kind of sickly glossy appearance. Secondly it becomes a breeding place for the causative agents of acnes and pimples to thrive unhindered **especially at night time.** The result?

Acne and pimples on the face.

And to worsen matters some began to use their fingers to press and break them. As they do this blood and a thick oily pus spurts out. As they spurts out a part of them is smeared on the face and a new generation of acne and pimples springs up there. Even a set of pimples larger in number than the former one from which the oily pus and blood spurted out. So what is the way out?

Just as sinus and phlegm secretion is necessary for lubrication of the respiratory tracts, over secretion of it due to imbalance in pressure in the body metabolism causes respiratory complaints like, catarrh, running nose and other sinus complications. In this situation, anti-semiotics like piriton and anti allergic drugs like loratin will be required to regulate and put things in check. So also is over secretion of oil in the face can be put in check and regulated to prevent and cure acnes and pimples.

But you don't need drugs here to regulate the secretions but some dietary and disciplinary measures.

1. If you have been cooking your soup with vegetable oil, stop and switch over to palm oil henceforth. Or if palm oil is not available in your place, try and be using OLIVE OIL for change. No matter the tribe where you came from, use palm oil for your cooking hence forth. I learnt that some tribes in the Northern Nigeria or some race in the some parts of the world don't cook their soups with palm oil but vegetable oils. Maybe due to non availability. Or rather, it is not readily or easily available.

To this group of people, if PALM OIL is not readily available in their area, I recommend OLIVE OIL for frying or seasoning their stews or soups until the 'trouble' on the face is over.

2.   My honest advice to any among them battling acnes and pimples to try palm oil for a change and discover how sweet and delicious it could be to cook with it of any delicacy.

To worsen matters some even use vegetable oils to first fry and cook 'egusi' (melon seeds!) as soup. And in a matter of days acnes and pimples will spring up like cocoa pods on their faces! Why won't they spring up? After all, a fallow and fertile ground has been cultivated for their growth. So **henceforth avoid as much as possible vegetable oil for now.** Use palm oil for all your cooking for now.

What of if you want to fry plantain you will say? Must you always eat fried plantain? Can't you deny yourself of it for now? And if you must eat fried plantain can't you be frying it with palm oil for now or olive oil? What of fried chicken? Can't you deny yourself of it for now? And if you must eat chicken, can't you eat it roasted for now? Could you now see where **self-control and self-denial comes in?**

3.   Found of nuts? I mean groundnuts? Stop it now until further notice. Be it to 'smoke' garri (switch to coconut or dry fish for a change), or to eat banana with or taking it ordinarily. Groundnuts are oily and will increase the intensity of the oil secretions from the pores. Just as phlegm secretion is to be regulated by the use of drugs in the case of sinus related diseases, so also must dietary regulations be used to check intensity of oil secretions on your face.

Bottomline? Knock out groundnuts and other oily nuts including cashew nuts from your diets until further notice. Again **self-denial and self-discipline is it.**

4.   Many like ponded yam and 'egusi' (melon seed)soup, to be stepped down with a bottle of larger at a restaurant. Egusi seed is very rich in oil and fats. To say it is oily is to make an understatement. In as much as we are regulating secretion of oils especially on your face, egusi comes under the hammer, even if you want to cook it with palm oil. Egusi means melon. Including a family member white melon seeds called 'itoos' by the Yorubas, eaten merely boiled by some and eaten in dried seed form by the Kabbas of Kogi State, all them avoid. Remember **self-discipline and self-denial.** In conclusion every oily seed must

be knocked out of your diets for now in cooked fried or raw form.

5.   What of magarines and butter? Of course, they are oily in nature, form and composition. And all we are doing is regulating oil secretion and generation on your face. So as one of the measures to achieve this, they have to leave your breakfast table **with immediate effect.** It is not because you are poor that you cannot afford to put margarines or butter on your table. Let whoever asks you questions about it know that you are checkmating acnes and pimples. If they mock or sneer, tell them they can hang for all you care. You need a smooth face. Can't you see mine on facebook? Smooth fresh and young like a twenty year old, yet I am in my late fourties.

6 WHEN BATHING

Each time you are in the bathroom to take your bath and you want to wash your face, never, never, never and I repeat **don't sponge your face.** Squeeze the soap in between your two palms severally; doing that will leave them messy with layers of soap from the bar. Now use those hands layered with soap to wash your face very well and rinse the lathers off your face. Don't worry, your face is clean. You don't need to apply sponge on your face before it can be clean washing. There are some who don't even apply sponge on their body when washing. All they do is lathering their body with the soap and rinse off and they are washed clean.

Squeezing your face with sponge scratches stimulates and sensitises the pores and in essence motivates acnes and pimples to come out. **Just as more rashes comes out of the body of a man with rashes when he keeps scratching them, sponging your face scratches it and keep the pimples flowing out.**

Again **self-discipline, self-control and self-denial is it.**

RESULTS NEVER COMES OVERNIGHT, BUT KEEP AT IT CONSISITENTLY FOR DAYS, WEEKS, MONTHS EVEN IF IT WILL TAKE YEARS.

NOW TO THE DOS

All said and done, measures have now been taken to regulate the inflow and outflow of oil on the face by taking some dietary measures. Let now come to the existing oils on the face that the microbes of acnes and pimples are feasting on, making your face a shadow of itself.

As a student of Public Health I have been taught in my basic studies days to understand that prevention is better and cheaper than cure. All I am offering in this information is a surer way of **preventing** and at the same time **stopping** acnes and pimples from making a basketball field out of your face which is far cheaper than having it and looking for expensive cures via facial treatments, lotions, taking blood purifier capsules, etc.etc.

The good news now is that if you are suffering from acnes and pimples, the information being shared here are both **curative and preventive measures.** May be you want **to know the guinea pig for the research that lead to the discovery of this information. It was no other person than my humble self.**

Necessity, the saying goes, is the mother of invention. I will share my testimony later when I want to conclude.

Let us go again into business.

There is nothing wrong in using any NAFDAC registered medicated soaps to wash yourself and your face when bathing. Just be very careful of the ones the quacks peddle in buses, 'molues' (name of rugged some rickety public buses in Nigeria) and road sides, lest you add fuel to the fire or add insult to injury or both. Again for the sake of emphasis **never sponge your face when bathing** be it in the night and daytime. Simply lather your face with the soap, toilet or medicated, and rinse.

For over 20 years I have never sponged my face when bathing and I have not become ugly or for it or but rather I developed a radiant baby like face, SMOOTH like a brook side stone.

Now it is night and you want to go to bed.

Many take showers before going to bed. I don't, not until my wife swore it is going to be over her dead body. Yet, when I was using myself as the experiment when I was very young in my twenties in the nineties, I will simply wash my face **at night** with a toilet or medicated soap, clean it a towel before applying the steps I will outline below with proven scientific explanations.

Having washed your face at night before going to bed with either toilet or medicated soap, wipe it clean and dry with a towel. This done, apply in large and generous quantity layers of **coloured talcum** (NOT WHITE MEDICATED) **powder** on your face until you look yourself in the mirror and look like a fetish priest. Then go to bed.

Make sure you have bid your neighbours good night and put your children to bed, if you are married and with children, and be sure you are seeing nobody again until the following morning after washing your face and applying this powder on your face. Otherwise whoever sees you after will either run for dear life, or dive for cover or raise alarm thinking he has seen a ghost or that something is wrong somewhere. Don't worry about your husband, he will understand. And if it is the man, your wife will understand though she may see it as funny and make a good laugh out it.

Let me repeat this for the sake of emphasis and clarity. Let the powder be a **SMOOTH coloured talcum powder** NOT **a white medicated powder**. It doesn't have to be an expensive one. It could be any of these medium priced ones readily available in the open market.

Just make sure it is a **coloured TALCUM** powder.

There was this brand of talcum powder called 'SWEET SIXTEEN'. That was what I used to apply on my face every night then. And within days I would have exhausted the tin because of the large quantities I apply every night. Then I will buy another one again.

Apply this powder on your face in such a way that you won't see any layer of your facial skin again except the colour of the powder all over your face. Then go to bed. When you wake up the following morning, go check up yourself before the mirror. You will discover that except for some little tiny very faint patches of traces of the powder, every layer of this powder has disappeared on your face and all you can see the real colour of your face now, hitherto covered the previous night by a thick layer of talcum powder!

So what happened to this powder you applied on your face overnight?

Answer: This is to tell you the enormity of oil your face secreted and generated through night, which these thick layers of coloured talcum powder drained off until it was overwhelmed and it disappeared on your face by the following morning.

Next question: Supposing you did not apply these layers of coloured talcum powder on your face and your face kept secreting and generating oil all through the night and there was nothing to drain this large quantity of oil on your face?

Answer: Then the causative agents of acne and pimples would have been having a field day, swimming freely and enjoying themselves on your face all through the night! And like a yam farmer from Benue State of Nigeria constructs ridges for yam, so these micro organisms would have constructed various size of ridges of pimples on your face!

Because these acnes and pimples causing micro agents thrive in the oily environment of an oily face!

Oil is the media on which they breed and multiply, just as bacteria that cause colds and pneumonia multiply at room temperature.

But when your face has been dried and drained of all oil with talcum powder and there is no oil on which they can feed and thrive on, they get starved of nutrients and air, suffocate and wither off from your face

at the end of the day. And this take several weeks and months, or years depending on the intensity of the acnes and pimples on the face. It will take that long because a famine victim did not die on the very first day of starvation. But after several days, and if it is that of a malnourished child, it may even take a year.

The same goes for the causative agents of acnes and pimples on your face.

But you can be sure that that you are now making life miserable for these agents of facial destruction, by malnourishing, starving and suffocating them of their food air – facial oils - and their withering away is a matter of time.

Each night they come and met your face dried with no oil on it for them to feed and thrive on; and these goes on for several

weeks and months even for over a year or years, they will suffocate and die of malnutrition, starvation and asphyxiation and leave your face alone and for good.

One thing I can guarantee you at the end of the day is that your face will be free of stubborn acnes and pimples, no matter how long it takes. And I don't need to give you a money back guarantee, because you will begin to see results within 2 weeks of consistent application of these remedies.

I can bet you that I am very sure.

With this, I can now tell my story.

As a lone bachelor in my apartment in Ogbomoso in present day Oyo State of Nigeria in 1988, my face infested with acnes and pimples. I have used all manner of medicated soap all to no avail. I have meanwhile kept away from oily foods and like vegetable oil, groundnuts, egusi (melon seed) soup, peanuts and margarines. But my oily face still remains a football field for these ugly micro-organisms at night and I was ignorant of what I am sharing with you now.

But there was this ragged half used tin of 'sweet sixteen' talcum powder lying fallow on my shelf, which I occasionally used thinly and lightly to freshen my face each time I am going out. I have been hearing of blood purifiers that when taken it will cleanse you inside out and rid you of the micro-organisms. But my budget cannot even accommodate going to a chemist to buy one. No thanks to my meagre pay as a civil servant then. All I do is bath with medicated soap every now and then.

So this night I came home. I cant really explain what came over as they says, curious idleness or trial and error, I took this tin talcum powder pour its contents on my generously in hands and applied thick layers of it on my face and went to bed. The following morning I discovered that all the powder is gone which somehow made me curious to try it again with the same result the following morning.

But what kept me doing this until I exhausted the tin of talcum powder and bought another one?

ANSWER: First it was curiosity. Secondly I discovered that every morning I look at myself in the mirror, my face becomes fresher after the previous night's application of talcum powder on it. So I want to enjoy looking at this freshness every morning and enjoy this while it lasted. I therefore kept doing it every night daily for weeks and months with even larger quantities of this powder and what I see each morning in the mirror dazzled me. Not only was my face looking fresher, it was getting smoother! Haba! So I kept at it for close to a year all through 1989 even to 1990 with fantastic results each morning!

Each time I exhausted a tin of talcum powder, I will throw the empty tin away and buy another one. And my facial appearance was getting not only fresher but younger. I did not even know when the pimples disappear. And the rest is now history. (Check my pictures on my wall on Facebook or let us meet physically to confirm)

Yet in my ignorance then, it never occurred to me that it was the oil on my face that the powder drains off each night I applied it, which in turn starved and suffocated the causative agents of acnes and pimples. Not until my background as Public Health professional lead me into further research and discoveries as to why these things are so.

NOW WHAT FINALLY HAPPENS TO THESE 'UNPRODUCTIVE' MICRO ORGANISMS?

When there is no oxygen for a mosquito larvae or pupae to breathe, no thanks to layers of oil applied on the water surface where they are breeding, they die and wither off.

The same applies to these micro organisms and bacteria when they have no oily surface on your face to breathe and play for days and months. They are **WEAKENED** wearied out, and they return to the body system, weak from starvation and suffocation. Then the red blood corpuscles, that constitutes the body defence system, by destroying disease causing micro organisms in the body find them **cheap and easy** preys in their weak state and destroy them! And in essence they get flushed out urine!

AND FINALLY THE GOOD NEWS?

Now I eat soups cooked with vegetable soup. I enjoy 'egusi' soup prepared with vegetable oil and as I am typing this I have just eaten an enormous quantity of groundnuts. I don't apply the powder at night because I don't even have a tin of it in the house. Yet my face has remained smooth, fresh and spotless ever since.

So where do we go from here as we conclude? All the DON'TS and DO above are two stones to kill a bird. Not a stone to kill two birds this time. But two stones of DON'TS and DOS to starve and suffocate the causative agents of acnes and pimples of facial oils, the media on which they thrive to perpetrate their heinous acts on your face.

Finally **your abstinence from these oily foods and nut in the DON'TS part are temporary not permanent** unlike in the case of sicknesses when a man or woman is banned from taking certain foods for life. Yours is temporary, as you can begin to enjoy back your fried plantains, egusi and groundnuts and any oily food after have gotten your face back, having ridden it of acnes and pimples.

www.ingramcontent.com/pod-product-compliance
Lightning Source LLC
Chambersburg PA
CBHW070254290526
45789CB00004B/1850